TABLE OF CONTENTS

Chapter 4: Diagnosis and Treatment

Screening for postpartum depression

Diagnosis of postpartum depression

Treatment options: medication, therapy, and self-care

Alternative and complementary treatments

Chapter 5: Coping with Postpartum Depression

Coping strategies for mothers

Coping strategies for partners and family members

Navigating the healthcare system

Support groups and resources

Chapter 6: Prevention and Early Intervention

Preventive measures for postpartum depression

Early intervention for at-risk mothers

Postpartum depression and subsequent pregnancies

Chapter 7: Personal Stories

Real-life stories of women who experienced postpartum depression

Lessons learned and advice for others

Chapter 8: Conclusion

The importance of addressing postpartum depression

Future directions for research and advocacy

INTRODUCTION

Motherhood is often depicted as a joyous and fulfilling experience, but the reality is that it can also be a challenging and overwhelming time. Postpartum depression is a common mental health issue that affects many new mothers, yet it is often overlooked and misunderstood.

This book aims to provide a comprehensive guide to postpartum depression, offering insight into the causes, symptoms, and treatment options for this condition.

In this book, we will explore the various biological, psychological, and social factors that can contribute to postpartum depression. We will also examine the emotional, behavioral, and physical symptoms of postpartum depression, as well as the impact it can have on mothers, infants, and families. Additionally, we will discuss the various treatment options available, including medication, therapy, self-care, and alternative and complementary treatments.

This book also includes real-life stories of women who have experienced postpartum depression, sharing their experiences and offering valuable insight into the challenges and successes of navigating this condition. Furthermore, we will provide advice and coping strategies for mothers, partners, and family members, as well as information on support groups and resources.

It is our hope that this book will provide a valuable resource for mothers and their

loved ones, as well as healthcare providers, policymakers, and anyone interested

in understanding and addressing postpartum depression. By raising awareness

and providing evidence-based information and support, we can work towards

improving the lives of mothers and families affected by postpartum depression.

Chapter 1: What really is Postpartum Depression

What is Postpartum Depression

Postpartum depression (PPD) is a type of depression that can occur in women after giving birth. It is a mood disorder that can affect a woman's emotions, thoughts, and behavior, and it can make it difficult for her to care for herself and her baby. PPD can occur anytime in the first year after childbirth, but it is most common within the first three months.

PPD can range from mild to severe and can last for weeks, months, or even longer if left untreated. Symptoms of PPD may include feelings of sadness, guilt, and hopelessness, changes in appetite and sleep patterns, loss of interest in activities, difficulty bonding with the baby, and thoughts of harming oneself or the baby. It is important to seek help if experiencing any of these symptoms, as PPD is a treatable condition with the right support and treatment.

Prevalence of Postpartum Depression

Postpartum depression (PPD) is a common and significant mental health condition that can occur in women after giving birth. It is estimated that between 10-20% of new mothers in the United States experience PPD, making it the most common complication of childbirth. However, the prevalence of PPD can vary depending on the study population, diagnostic criteria, and cultural factors.

Globally, studies have shown that the prevalence of PPD varies widely, ranging from 6% to as high as 40%. The incidence of PPD may be affected by cultural factors such as differences in social support, stigma, and healthcare access. For example, studies have found that immigrant women and women from certain cultures may be at higher risk of PPD due to acculturation stress, language barriers, and discrimination.

In addition, certain risk factors can increase the likelihood of developing PPD. These factors may include a personal or family history of depression or anxiety, a difficult or traumatic childbirth experience, a lack of social support, financial stress, and hormonal changes.

PPD can have significant consequences for both the mother and her child. It can interfere with the mother's ability to care for herself and her baby, negatively affect maternal-infant bonding, and increase the risk of long-term mental health problems. In addition, PPD can have an impact on the father and other family members, who may experience stress and anxiety as they try to support the mother and her baby.

It is important to recognize the signs and symptoms of PPD and seek help if experiencing them. Treatment options for PPD may include talk therapy, medication, self-care strategies, and support groups.

Myths and Misconceptions about Postpartum Depression

There are many myths and misconceptions about postpartum depression (PPD) that can prevent women from seeking help and can contribute to stigma and shame. Here are some common myths and misconceptions about PPD:

Myth: PPD is just a normal part of motherhood.
Reality: PPD is a serious medical condition that requires treatment. While many women experience some mood changes after childbirth, PPD is more severe and can interfere with a woman's ability to care for herself and her baby.

Myth: PPD only happens to women who have a history of depression.
Reality: While having a history of depression or anxiety can increase the risk of developing PPD, it can affect any woman, regardless of her mental health history.

Myth: PPD only happens immediately after childbirth.

Reality: While PPD often develops within the first few months after childbirth, it can occur anytime within the first year. In some cases, PPD may not develop until several months after childbirth.

Myth: PPD is caused by a lack of maternal instincts or bonding with the baby.

Reality: PPD is a medical condition that is caused by a combination of factors, including hormonal changes, stress, and genetic predisposition. It is not a result of a woman's ability to bond with her baby.

Myth: PPD is a sign of weakness or personal failure.

Reality: PPD is not a sign of weakness or personal failure. It is a medical condition that can affect anyone and requires treatment.

Myth: PPD only affects women.

Reality: While PPD is more common in women, men can also experience postpartum depression or anxiety. Studies have shown that up to 1 in 10 new fathers experience symptoms of PPD.

It is important to recognize and dispel these myths and misconceptions about PPD in order to increase awareness and reduce stigma. PPD is a treatable condition, and seeking help is an important step towards recovery.vention and treatment can help reduce the severity and duration of symptoms and improve outcomes for both the mother and her baby.

Overall, PPD is a significant public health issue that requires increased awareness, research, and resources to improve prevention, diagnosis, and treatment.

Chapter 2: Causes and Risk Factors

Biological factors of Postpartum Depression

Postpartum depression (PPD) is a complex disorder with many potential causes, including biological, psychological, and social factors. Here are some of the biological factors that have been identified as potential contributors to PPD:

Hormonal changes: During pregnancy, a woman's body undergoes significant hormonal changes, including increased levels of estrogen, progesterone, and cortisol. After childbirth, these hormone levels drop dramatically, which can contribute to mood changes and PPD.

Genetics: PPD may have a genetic component, as studies have shown that women with a family history of depression or anxiety are more likely to experience PPD. In addition, certain genes that are involved in regulating mood and stress responses may also play a role.

Neurotransmitters: Neurotransmitters are chemicals in the brain that regulate mood and other functions. Changes in the levels or function of certain neurotransmitters, such as serotonin and dopamine, have been linked to depression, including PPD.

Inflammation: Inflammation is a natural response to injury or infection, but chronic inflammation has been linked to a variety of health problems, including depression. Studies have found that women with PPD may have higher levels of inflammation markers in their blood.

Sleep disturbances: Sleep disruptions are common in new mothers, and sleep deprivation has been linked to mood changes and depression. In addition, disruptions to the body's circadian rhythm, or internal clock, can also contribute to PPD.

It is important to note that PPD is likely caused by a combination of biological, psychological, and social factors, and the exact cause may vary from woman to woman. However, understanding the biological factors that may contribute to PPD can help with prevention and treatment efforts. Hormonal therapies, antidepressant medications, and psychotherapy may all be effective in treating PPD, depending on the underlying causes and severity of symptoms.

Psychological factors of Postpartum Depression

In addition to biological factors, there are also several psychological factors that can contribute to postpartum depression (PPD). Here are some examples:

History of depression or anxiety: Women who have a history of depression or anxiety are more likely to experience PPD. This may be due to a combination of genetic, biological, and environmental factors.

Stressful life events: Stressful life events, such as financial difficulties, relationship problems, or health problems, can increase the risk of developing PPD. The stress of adjusting to a new baby, lack of sleep, and changes in routine can also contribute to PPD.

Lack of social support: Women who lack social support, such as a partner, family, or friends, may be more vulnerable to PPD. Social support can provide emotional and practical help, which can be especially important during the early postpartum period.

Perfectionism and unrealistic expectations: Women who have high expectations for themselves or their baby, or who strive for perfection, may be more likely to experience PPD. The reality of motherhood can be challenging and messy, and it can be difficult to live up to the idealized image of the "perfect mother".

Poor self-esteem: Women who struggle with low self-esteem, negative self-talk, or feelings of inadequacy may be more susceptible to PPD. The challenges of motherhood can trigger feelings of self-doubt and negative self-evaluation.

Traumatic childbirth experience: Women who have had a traumatic childbirth experience, such as a difficult delivery or complications during pregnancy, may be at higher risk for PPD. Traumatic experiences can trigger feelings of fear, anxiety, and depression.

It is important to note that these psychological factors can interact with biological factors to contribute to the development of PPD. Understanding the psychological factors that can contribute to PPD can help with prevention and treatment efforts. Psychotherapy, support groups, and stress-reduction techniques may all be effective in treating PPD, depending on the underlying causes and severity of symptoms.

Social and Cultural Factors of Postpartum Depression

Social and cultural factors can also play a role in the development of postpartum depression (PPD). Here are some examples:

Social support: Lack of social support, such as a lack of help with household chores or childcare, can contribute to PPD. This may be particularly true for women who lack support from their partner, family, or friends.

Cultural expectations: Cultural expectations about motherhood and gender roles can also play a role in PPD. For example, some cultures may place a greater emphasis on motherhood as a woman's primary role, which can contribute to feelings of inadequacy or guilt if a woman feels she is not living up to these expectations.

Stigma and shame: Stigma and shame surrounding mental health issues, including PPD, can make it more difficult for women to seek help. This can be especially true in cultures where mental illness is stigmatized or where there is a perception that seeking help for mental health issues is a sign of weakness.

Economic status: Economic stressors, such as financial difficulties or lack of access to affordable healthcare, can contribute to PPD. Women who are struggling to make ends meet may have less access to resources and support that can help alleviate the stress of motherhood.

Race and ethnicity: Research has shown that women of color may be at higher risk for PPD due to systemic factors such as racism, discrimination, and lack of access to healthcare. Additionally, cultural factors such as differences in beliefs about mental health and healthcare can impact the likelihood of seeking treatment for PPD.

Immigration status: Women who are immigrants or refugees may be at higher risk for PPD due to factors such as language barriers, lack of social support, and experiences of trauma related to displacement.

Understanding the social and cultural factors that can contribute to PPD is important for healthcare providers and support systems to provide culturally responsive care and support. Women may benefit from culturally sensitive counseling, peer support groups, and community resources that address their unique needs and circumstances.

Medical conditions that can mimic Postpartum Depression

There are several medical conditions that can mimic or contribute to symptoms of postpartum depression (PPD). It is important for healthcare providers to rule out these conditions before diagnosing PPD, as treatment may differ depending on the underlying cause. Here are some examples:

Thyroid disorders: Thyroid disorders, such as hypothyroidism or hyperthyroidism, can cause symptoms similar to those of PPD, including fatigue, irritability, and difficulty sleeping. Blood tests can determine if a woman has a thyroid disorder, and treatment may include medication to regulate thyroid hormone levels.

Anemia: Anemia, a condition in which there is a deficiency of red blood cells, can cause symptoms such as fatigue, weakness, and difficulty concentrating. Anemia is common in pregnancy and postpartum, and iron supplements or dietary changes may be recommended to address the deficiency.

Sleep disorders: Sleep disorders, such as sleep apnea or insomnia, can contribute to symptoms of PPD. Lack of sleep can exacerbate feelings of depression and anxiety. Treatment may involve lifestyle changes, such as improving sleep hygiene or using a continuous positive airway pressure (CPAP) machine for sleep apnea.

Chronic pain: Chronic pain, such as back pain or pelvic pain, can contribute to symptoms of depression and anxiety. Women who are experiencing chronic pain postpartum should be evaluated by a healthcare provider to determine the underlying cause and appropriate treatment.

Substance use disorders: Substance use disorders, such as alcohol or drug abuse, can mimic symptoms of PPD. Women who are struggling with substance use postpartum should be referred to addiction treatment services.

Neurological conditions: Certain neurological conditions, such as multiple sclerosis or epilepsy, can contribute to symptoms of depression and anxiety. Women who are experiencing neurological symptoms postpartum should be evaluated by a healthcare provider to determine the underlying cause and appropriate treatment.

It is important for healthcare providers to conduct a thorough evaluation of a woman's physical health in addition to her mental health when assessing for postpartum depression. Addressing any underlying medical conditions can improve outcomes for both the mother and baby.

Chapter 3: SYMPTOMS OF POSTPARTUM DEPRESSION

Emotional symptoms of postpartum depression

Persistent sadness or feelings of hopelessness: Women with PPD may feel sad or overwhelmed for most of the day, every day. They may also feel hopeless about their ability to feel better or cope with their symptoms.

Anxiety or excessive worry: Women with PPD may feel anxious or worried about their baby's health, their own health, or their ability to care for their baby. They may have intrusive thoughts or images that cause them to feel more anxious.

Irritability or anger: Women with PPD may feel more irritable than usual, and may snap at loved ones or become easily frustrated. They may also feel angry or resentful towards their baby or partner.

Loss of interest or pleasure: Women with PPD may lose interest in activities that they previously enjoyed, such as hobbies or spending time with friends. They may also have difficulty bonding with their baby or feel a sense of detachment.

Guilt or shame: Women with PPD may feel guilty or ashamed about their symptoms, and may feel like they are a bad mother or not living up to their own or others' expectations.

Difficulty concentrating or making decisions: Women with PPD may have difficulty concentrating, remembering things, or making decisions. They may feel like their mind is in a fog.

Thoughts of self-harm or suicide: In severe cases of PPD, women may have thoughts of self-harm or suicide. It is important to seek immediate medical attention if these thoughts occur.

If you or someone you know is experiencing any of these emotional symptoms postpartum, it is important to seek help from a healthcare provider or mental health professional. Treatment for PPD may include counseling, medication, or a combination of both. With appropriate treatment, most women with PPD can recover and enjoy a healthy and fulfilling relationship with their baby.

Behavioral Symptoms of Postpartum Depression

Postpartum depression (PPD) can also cause a range of behavioral symptoms that can interfere with a mother's ability to care for herself and her baby. Here are some common behavioral symptoms of PPD:

Withdrawing from loved ones: Women with PPD may withdraw from family and friends, and may isolate themselves from others. They may feel like they are a burden or that others won't understand what they are going through.

Neglecting personal care: Women with PPD may neglect their own self-care, such as showering, eating well, or getting enough rest. They may also neglect their baby's care, such as missing doctor's appointments or not responding to the baby's needs.

Changes in appetite or weight: Women with PPD may experience changes in appetite or weight, such as eating too much or too little, or gaining or losing weight rapidly.

Insomnia or excessive sleeping: Women with PPD may have difficulty sleeping, even when the baby is sleeping, or may sleep excessively and have difficulty waking up.

Using alcohol or drugs: Women with PPD may use alcohol or drugs to cope with their symptoms, which can make their depression worse and interfere with their ability to care for their baby.

Experiencing physical symptoms: Women with PPD may experience physical symptoms such as headaches, stomachaches, or muscle tension.

Avoiding the baby: Women with PPD may avoid interacting with their baby, or may feel overwhelmed by the baby's needs. They may also have difficulty bonding with the baby.

It is important to seek help from a healthcare provider or mental health professional if you or someone you know is experiencing any of these behavioral symptoms postpartum. Treatment for PPD may include counseling, medication, or a combination of both. With appropriate treatment, most women with PPD can recover and enjoy a healthy and fulfilling relationship with their baby.

Physical symptoms of Postpartum depression

Postpartum depression (PPD) can also cause a range of physical symptoms. While these symptoms can be caused by other medical conditions as well, they can be a sign of PPD when experienced in combination with emotional and behavioral symptoms. Here are some common physical symptoms of PPD:

Fatigue: Women with PPD may feel extremely tired, even after getting enough sleep. They may also have difficulty staying awake during the day.

Headaches or body aches: Women with PPD may experience headaches or body aches, such as muscle tension or pain.

Digestive problems: Women with PPD may experience digestive problems such as constipation, diarrhea, or nausea.

Changes in appetite: Women with PPD may experience changes in appetite, such as loss of appetite or overeating.

Sleep problems: Women with PPD may have difficulty falling asleep or staying asleep, or may sleep excessively.

Physical agitation or restlessness: Women with PPD may experience physical agitation or restlessness, such as pacing, fidgeting, or tapping.

Decreased libido: Women with PPD may experience a decrease in their sex drive.

It is important to seek help from a healthcare provider or mental health professional if you or someone you know is experiencing any of these physical symptoms postpartum. Treatment for PPD may include counseling, medication, or a combination of both. With appropriate treatment, most women with PPD can recover and enjoy a healthy and fulfilling relationship with their baby.

Postpartum psychosis

Postpartum psychosis is a rare but serious mental health condition that can occur in some women after giving birth. It typically begins within the first two weeks after delivery and is considered a medical emergency, as it can lead to thoughts of harm towards the mother or baby.

Symptoms of postpartum psychosis can include:

- Confusion or disorientation
- Hallucinations (seeing or hearing things that are not there)
- Delusions (having beliefs that are not based in reality)
- Paranoia or suspicion
- Rapid mood swings
- Agitation or irritability
- Inability to sleep or excessive sleeping

- Inappropriate behavior

Postpartum psychosis is considered a medical emergency, and women who experience these symptoms should seek immediate medical attention. Treatment may include hospitalization, medication, and therapy.

It is important to note that postpartum psychosis is different from postpartum depression, although both can occur after childbirth. While postpartum depression is a common and treatable condition that can last for several weeks or months, postpartum psychosis is much less common and requires immediate medical attention.

Chapter 4: Diagnosis and Treatment

Screening for postpartum depression

Screening for postpartum depression involves using specific tools to identify women who may be experiencing symptoms of depression after giving birth. These tools are typically questionnaires that women can fill out either at their postpartum check-up or on their own. The screening tools ask questions about symptoms of depression, anxiety, and other emotional and behavioral changes that can oHere are some common screening tools used to identify PPD:

Edinburgh Postnatal Depression Scale (EPDS): The EPDS is a commonly used self-report screening tool that asks women to rate their experience of depression symptoms over the past week. It includes questions about mood, anxiety, guilt, sleep, and appetite.

Postpartum Depression Screening Scale (PDSS): The PDSS is another self-report screening tool that assesses women's experience of depression symptoms over the past week, as well as their anxiety, stress, and adjustment to motherhood.

Patient Health Questionnaire-9 (PHQ-9): The PHQ-9 is a self-report screening tool that assesses depression symptoms over the past two weeks. It includes questions about mood, sleep, appetite, and concentration.

Beck Depression Inventory (BDI): The BDI is a self-report screening tool that assesses depression symptoms over the past week. It includes questions about mood, pessimism, guilt, and self-esteem.

General Practitioner Assessment of Cognition (GPCOG): The GPCOG is a screening tool that assesses cognitive function in older adults, but it has also been used to screen for cognitive impairment in postpartum women that occur after childbirth.

The Edinburgh Postnatal Depression Scale (EPDS), Postpartum Depression Screening Scale (PDSS), Patient Health Questionnaire-9 (PHQ-9), Beck Depression Inventory (BDI), and General Practitioner Assessment of Cognition (GPCOG) are all examples of screening tools that can be used to identify PPD. Each tool has its own set of questions and scoring system, but they all aim to identify women who may be experiencing symptoms of depression.

It is important to note that screening is not a diagnosis of postpartum depression, but rather a way to identify women who may be at risk and require further evaluation and treatment. Healthcare providers can use the results of the screening tools to initiate a conversation with the woman about her symptoms and provide appropriate support and treatment, such as counseling, medication, or both.

Overall, screening for postpartum depression is an important part of maternal healthcare, as it can help identify women who may be struggling with emotional and behavioral changes after giving birth and provide them with the help they need.

Diagnosis of postpartum depression

Diagnosing postpartum depression (PPD) involves a thorough evaluation by a healthcare professional, typically a mental health provider or primary care physician. There is no specific test for PPD, so the diagnosis is usually based on a combination of the woman's reported symptoms, her medical history, and her healthcare provider's observations.

To diagnose PPD, healthcare providers typically use the criteria from the Diagnostic and Statistical Manual of Mental Disorders (DSM-5), which is a standard reference used by mental health professionals. According to the DSM-5, to be diagnosed with PPD, a woman must experience five or more of the following symptoms nearly every day for at least two weeks:

- Depressed mood most of the day, nearly every day
- Markedly diminished interest or pleasure in activities nearly every day
- Significant weight loss when not dieting or weight gain or decrease or increase in appetite
- Insomnia or hypersomnia nearly every day
- Psychomotor agitation or retardation nearly every day
- Fatigue or loss of energy nearly every day
- Feelings of worthlessness or excessive or inappropriate guilt nearly every day
- Diminished ability to think or concentrate, or indecisiveness, nearly every day
- Recurrent thoughts of death, recurrent suicidal ideation without a specific plan, or a suicide attempt or a specific plan for committing suicide

To be diagnosed with PPD, these symptoms must cause significant distress or impairment in social, occupational, or other important areas of functioning.

It is important to note that healthcare providers may also consider other factors, such as the woman's medical history, family history of mental health disorders, and current stressors, when making a diagnosis of PPD.

If a woman is diagnosed with PPD, she may be referred to a mental health provider for further evaluation and treatment, which may include therapy, medication, or both.

Treatment options: medication, therapy, and self-care

Postpartum depression (PPD) is a serious mental health condition that affects some women after giving birth. It is estimated that up to 1 in 7 women experience PPD, making it one of the most common complications of childbirth. PPD can have a significant impact on a woman's quality of life and her ability to care for herself and her baby. However, with the right treatment and support, most women with PPD can recover and enjoy motherhood.

There are several treatment options available for PPD, including medication, therapy, and self-care practices. Medication, such as antidepressants, can be effective in reducing symptoms of depression, anxiety, and sleep problems. However, it is important for women to discuss the risks and benefits of medication with their healthcare provider, especially if they are breastfeeding.

Therapy, or talk therapy, can also be effective in treating PPD. Cognitive-behavioral therapy (CBT) is a type of therapy that helps women identify and change negative thought patterns and behaviors that contribute to their depression. Interpersonal therapy (IPT) is another type of therapy that focuses on improving communication skills and interpersonal relationships. Therapy can also provide a safe and supportive environment for women to express their feelings and concerns.

Self-care practices, such as exercise, healthy eating, mindfulness, and social support, can also be helpful in managing PPD. Engaging in activities that promote relaxation and stress reduction, such as yoga or meditation, can help women feel more grounded and centered. Eating a balanced diet and staying physically active can also improve mood and energy levels. Social support, whether from family, friends, or a support group, can also provide a source of comfort and encouragement for women with PPD.

It is important to note that treatment for PPD is often multifaceted and may involve a combination of medication, therapy, and self-care practices. Women with PPD should work closely with their healthcare provider to develop a treatment plan that is tailored to their individual needs and preferences. Support from family and friends can also be invaluable in helping women with PPD navigate this challenging time.

If you or someone you know is experiencing symptoms of PPD, it is important to seek help from a healthcare provider. With proper treatment and support, women with PPD can fully recover and enjoy motherhood.

Alternative and complementary treatments

Alternative and complementary treatments may also be used to manage symptoms of postpartum depression (PPD). While these treatments have not been extensively studied or proven effective in clinical trials, some women may find them helpful in conjunction with other forms of treatment. Here are some examples:

Acupuncture: This is a traditional Chinese medicine technique that involves inserting thin needles into specific points on the body. Acupuncture may help improve mood, reduce anxiety, and promote relaxation.

Massage therapy: Massage therapy can help reduce muscle tension and promote relaxation. It can also improve sleep quality and reduce anxiety.

Herbal supplements: Some herbal supplements, such as St. John's wort, may have antidepressant effects. However, it is important to discuss the use of herbal supplements with a healthcare provider, as they may interact with other medications or have potential side effects.

Light therapy: Light therapy involves exposure to bright light, typically through a special lamp, and may help improve mood and reduce symptoms of depression.

Omega-3 fatty acids: Omega-3 fatty acids, found in fish oil and other sources, may have mood-stabilizing effects and help reduce symptoms of depression.

It is important to note that alternative and complementary treatments should not be used as a substitute for evidence-based treatment, such as medication and therapy. Women with PPD should discuss any alternative or complementary treatments with their healthcare provider and should not stop or change their prescribed treatment without first consulting their healthcare provider.

Chapter 5: Coping with Postpartum Depression

Coping strategies for mothers

Coping with postpartum depression (PPD) can be challenging, but there are many coping strategies that can help women manage their symptoms and improve their overall well-being. Here are some coping strategies that mothers with PPD may find helpful:

Reach out for support: It is important to reach out to family, friends, and healthcare providers for support. Joining a support group or connecting with other mothers who have experienced PPD can also be helpful.

Practice self-care: Taking care of oneself is important when dealing with PPD. This can include engaging in activities that promote relaxation, such as taking a warm bath or practicing yoga, eating a healthy diet, and getting regular exercise.

Get enough sleep: Lack of sleep can worsen symptoms of depression. Mothers should try to get enough sleep by taking naps when their baby is sleeping and asking for help from family or friends to care for their baby at night.

Seek professional help: It is important to seek professional help if symptoms of PPD persist or worsen. Healthcare providers can provide support, guidance, and effective treatments such as medication and therapy.

Break tasks into manageable steps: It can be overwhelming to take care of a new baby when experiencing PPD. Mothers can break tasks into smaller, more manageable steps, and focus on completing one task at a time.

Set realistic expectations: It is important to set realistic expectations for oneself when dealing with PPD. Mothers should not feel pressured to meet societal or personal expectations of motherhood and should focus on doing what is best for themselves and their baby.

Focus on positive self-talk: Negative self-talk can worsen symptoms of depression. Mothers should try to focus on positive self-talk and challenge negative thoughts.

Coping with PPD can be challenging, but with the right support, self-care, and professional help, mothers can recover and enjoy motherhood. It is important to remember that seeking help is a sign of strength, and there is no shame in experiencing PPD.

Coping strategies for partners and family members

Partners and family members can play a crucial role in supporting mothers who are experiencing postpartum depression (PPD). Here are some coping strategies for partners and family members:

Educate yourself about PPD: It is important to educate yourself about PPD so you can understand what your loved one is going through. This can also help you provide better support.

Offer practical help: Offer to help with household chores, cooking, and caring for the baby. This can help reduce stress for the mother and allow her to focus on self-care and recovery.

Encourage self-care: Encourage the mother to engage in activities that promote relaxation and self-care, such as taking a warm bath, getting a massage, or practicing yoga.

Listen without judgment: It is important to listen to the mother without judgment and provide a safe and supportive space for her to express her feelings.

Be patient: Recovery from PPD can take time, and it is important to be patient and supportive throughout the process.

Seek professional help: Encourage the mother to seek professional help if symptoms of PPD persist or worsen. Offer to help find a healthcare provider or accompany her to appointments.

Take care of yourself: Caring for a loved one with PPD can be challenging, and it is important to take care of yourself as well. This can include seeking your own support, practicing self-care, and taking breaks when needed.

It is important to remember that supporting a loved one with PPD can be difficult, and it is okay to feel overwhelmed or unsure of how to help. Seeking guidance from healthcare providers, support groups, or mental health professionals can also be helpful for partners and family members.

Navigating the healthcare system

Navigating the healthcare system can be challenging, especially when dealing with postpartum depression (PPD). Here are some tips for navigating the healthcare system when seeking help for PPD:

- Find a healthcare provider: The first step in seeking help for PPD is to find a healthcare provider who specializes in maternal mental health. This can include a psychiatrist, psychologist, or licensed clinical social worker.

- Ask for recommendations: Ask for recommendations from friends, family, or other healthcare providers, such as your obstetrician or pediatrician.

- Check with insurance: Check with your insurance provider to ensure that the healthcare provider you choose is covered under your insurance plan.

- Prepare for appointments: Prepare for appointments by writing down any symptoms you are experiencing, any questions you have, and any medications you are currently taking.

- Be honest and open: It is important to be honest and open with your healthcare provider about your symptoms and how you are feeling. This can help your provider develop an effective treatment plan.

- Advocate for yourself: If you feel that your concerns are not being addressed, or if you are not comfortable with the treatment plan, it is important to advocate for yourself and ask for a second opinion or seek a different healthcare provider.

- Seek support: Seek support from friends, family, or support groups when navigating the healthcare system. This can help reduce stress and provide a supportive community during the recovery process.

Navigating the healthcare system can be overwhelming, but with the right support and resources, mothers can receive the help they need to recover from PPD. It is important to remember that seeking help is a sign of strength, and there is no shame in experiencing PPD.

Support groups and resources

Support groups and resources can be valuable for mothers who are experiencing postpartum depression (PPD). Here are some options:

- Postpartum Support International: Postpartum Support International is a non-profit organization that provides resources and support for women experiencing perinatal mood and anxiety disorders, including PPD. They offer a helpline, online support groups, and a directory of healthcare providers.

- Local support groups: Many communities have local support groups for mothers with PPD. These groups can provide a safe and supportive space to share experiences and receive emotional support.

- Therapy: Therapy can be a valuable resource for mothers with PPD. Therapists who specialize in maternal mental health can provide individual or group therapy to help mothers address and cope with PPD symptoms.

- Online resources: There are many online resources available for mothers with PPD, including websites, forums, and apps. These resources can provide information, support, and guidance on coping strategies and treatment options.

- Family and friends: Family and friends can be a valuable source of support for mothers with PPD. Loved ones can offer emotional support, practical help, and encouragement during the recovery process.

- Healthcare providers: Healthcare providers can offer guidance and support for mothers with PPD. They can provide medical treatment, refer mothers to therapy or support groups, and monitor symptoms to ensure effective treatment.

It is important to remember that seeking help is a sign of strength, and mothers with PPD should not feel ashamed or alone. There are many resources available to support mothers during the recovery process, and with the right support and resources, mothers can recover and thrive.

Chapter 6: Prevention and Early Intervention

Preventive measures for postpartum depression

While postpartum depression (PPD) cannot always be prevented, there are steps that mothers can take to reduce the risk of developing PPD. Here are some preventive measures:

- Exercise: Exercise can help reduce stress and improve mood. Even moderate exercise, such as walking or yoga, can be beneficial.

- Self-care: It is important for mothers to prioritize self-care after giving birth. This can include getting enough sleep, eating a healthy diet, and taking time for activities that bring joy and relaxation.

- Support system: Building a strong support system of family, friends, and healthcare providers can help reduce stress and provide emotional support during the postpartum period.

- Education: Educating oneself about PPD can help reduce stigma and provide a better understanding of the condition. This can help mothers recognize symptoms and seek help if needed.

- Talk to healthcare providers: It is important for mothers to talk to their healthcare providers about any concerns or symptoms they may be experiencing. Healthcare providers can offer guidance, support, and treatment if needed.

- Consider therapy: Mothers who have a history of depression or who are experiencing significant stress or anxiety during pregnancy may benefit from therapy. Therapy can help address underlying issues and provide coping strategies.

- Medication: In some cases, medication may be recommended to prevent or treat PPD. Mothers should talk to their healthcare providers about the risks and benefits of medication during pregnancy and breastfeeding.

While there is no guaranteed way to prevent PPD, taking proactive steps can help reduce the risk and promote emotional well-being during the postpartum period.

Early intervention for at-risk mothers

Early intervention for at-risk mothers is important to prevent or minimize the impact of postpartum depression (PPD). Here are some early intervention strategies:

- Screening: Healthcare providers can screen mothers for PPD symptoms during pregnancy and postpartum visits. Screening can help identify at-risk mothers and provide early intervention and treatment.

- Education: Healthcare providers can provide education on PPD and its symptoms, as well as resources for support and treatment.

-

- Counseling: Counseling during pregnancy or postpartum can help mothers address underlying issues and develop coping strategies to prevent PPD.

- Medication: In some cases, medication may be recommended to prevent or treat PPD. Healthcare providers can discuss the risks and benefits of medication during pregnancy and breastfeeding.

- Support groups: Support groups for pregnant women and new mothers can provide emotional support and a safe space to share experiences and concerns.

- Family support: Family members can offer practical support, such as help with childcare or household tasks, to reduce stress and prevent PPD.

- Partner involvement: Partners can play a key role in early intervention by offering emotional support, helping with childcare, and encouraging mothers to seek treatment if needed.

Early intervention is crucial for at-risk mothers to prevent or minimize the impact of PPD. Healthcare providers, family members, and partners can all play a role in identifying and addressing PPD symptoms and providing support and resources for treatment.

Postpartum depression and subsequent pregnancies

Postpartum depression (PPD) can have an impact on subsequent pregnancies. Here are some ways PPD can affect subsequent pregnancies:

- Increased risk of PPD: Mothers who have experienced PPD in a previous pregnancy are at a higher risk of developing PPD in subsequent pregnancies.

- Increased risk of other mental health issues: Mothers who have experienced PPD may be at a higher risk of developing other mental health issues, such as anxiety or bipolar disorder, in subsequent pregnancies.

- Pregnancy complications: Mothers with a history of PPD may be at a higher risk of pregnancy complications, such as preterm birth or low birth weight.

- Impact on parenting: PPD can have an impact on a mother's ability to parent, which can affect subsequent pregnancies and the health and well-being of the child.

- Treatment considerations: Mothers with a history of PPD should discuss treatment options with their healthcare provider before becoming pregnant. Some medications used to treat PPD may not be safe during pregnancy or breastfeeding.

It is important for mothers with a history of PPD to discuss their experiences and concerns with their healthcare provider before becoming pregnant. Healthcare providers can provide support, education, and treatment options to help manage symptoms and promote emotional well-being during subsequent pregnancies.

Chapter 7: Personal Stories

Denise Welch: Actress and television presenter Denise Welch has spoken openly about her experience with postpartum depression after the birth of her son in 1990. She has described the intense feelings of sadness and despair she experienced, as well as the difficulty of coping with her symptoms while also caring for her newborn. She also highlighted the support of her Partner and family at that time. Denise Welch talked about it extensively in her book "pulling myself together"

Welch has been an advocate for mental health awareness and has used her platform to raise awareness about postpartum depression and the importance of seeking help. She has also shared her story to encourage other women who may be struggling to speak up and seek support.

Alanis Morissette: Singer-songwriter Alanis Morissette has spoken about her experience with postpartum depression after the birth of her son in 2010. She has been open about the intense anxiety and feelings of isolation she experienced, and how therapy and medication helped her manage her symptoms.

Drew Barrymore: Actress and producer Drew Barrymore has also been open about her struggles with postpartum depression after the birth of her second daughter in 2014. She has spoken about the importance of seeking help and the impact that therapy and self-care can have on mental health.

Gwyneth Paltrow: Actress and entrepreneur Gwyneth Paltrow has spoken about her experience with postpartum depression after the birth of her son in 2006. She has been open about the feelings of sadness and detachment she experienced, and how therapy and self-care helped her manage her symptoms.

Lisa Abramson: Lisa Abramson is a business coach and mental health advocate who has spoken about her experience with postpartum psychosis after the birth of her daughter in 2014. She has shared her story to raise awareness about the severity of postpartum mental health issues and the importance of early intervention.

Adele Geras: Adele Geras is a British author who wrote a book, "Facing the Light," about her experience with postpartum depression after the birth of her daughter in 1988. She has spoken about the stigma surrounding mental health issues at the time, and how writing about her experience helped her heal and connect with others.

Chrissy Teigen: Model and TV personality Chrissy Teigen has been open about her experience with postpartum depression after the birth of her daughter in 2016. She has spoken about the guilt and shame she felt, and how therapy and medication helped her manage her symptoms.

Adele: Grammy-winning singer Adele has also been open about her experience with postpartum depression after the birth of her son in 2012. She has spoken about how difficult it was to admit she needed help, but how therapy and the support of her partner helped her manage her symptoms.

Hayden Panettiere: Actress Hayden Panettiere has been open about her struggles with postpartum depression after the birth of her daughter in 2014. She has spoken about the importance of seeking help and the stigma surrounding mental health issues.

Brooke Shields: Actress and model Brooke Shields wrote a book, "Down Came the Rain: My Journey Through Postpartum Depression," about her experience with postpartum depression after the birth of her daughter in 2003. She has since become an advocate for mental health awareness and has spoken about the need for support and treatment for mothers with PPD.

Serena Williams: Tennis superstar Serena Williams has also been open about her experience with postpartum depression after the birth of her daughter in 2017. She has spoken about the challenges of being a new mother and a professional athlete, and the importance of seeking help and support.

These women's stories show that postpartum depression and related mental health issues can affect anyone, regardless of their background or circumstances. They also highlight the importance of seeking help, getting treatment, and raising awareness about postpartum mental health issues. By sharing their experiences, these women have helped to reduce the stigma surrounding mental health issues and promote understanding and support for mothers who may be struggling.

Here are some lessons learned and advice for others based on the experiences of women who have struggled with postpartum depression:

Seek help early: Many women who have experienced postpartum depression have emphasized the importance of seeking help as soon as possible. This may include reaching out to a healthcare provider, therapist, or support group for help managing symptoms and getting the necessary treatment.

Practice self-care: Taking care of yourself is crucial when dealing with postpartum depression. This may include getting enough rest, eating well, exercising, and engaging in activities that bring you joy and relaxation. It's important to prioritize self-care even when it feels difficult or overwhelming.

Connect with others: Many women have found support and comfort in connecting with others who have experienced postpartum depression or other mental health issues. This may include joining a support group, talking to a trusted friend or family member, or seeking out online resources and forums for support.

Be open and honest: Sharing your experience with postpartum depression with others can be a difficult and vulnerable process, but many women have found that it can also be incredibly healing and empowering. Being open and honest about your struggles can help reduce feelings of isolation and stigma, and may inspire others to seek help and support as well.

Remember that recovery is possible: While postpartum depression can be a challenging and difficult experience, it's important to remember that recovery is possible with the right treatment and support. Many women who have experienced postpartum depression have gone on to thrive and lead fulfilling lives with their families and loved ones. With time, patience, and the right

support, it is possible to overcome this challenging experience.

Chapter 8: Conclusion

The importance of addressing postpartum depression

Addressing postpartum depression is important for several reasons:

- Maternal and infant health: Postpartum depression can have a significant impact on both maternal and infant health. Untreated postpartum depression can lead to a range of negative health outcomes for both the mother and child, including developmental delays, difficulties with bonding and attachment, and increased risk of chronic health conditions.

- Family functioning: Postpartum depression can also have a significant impact on family functioning. It can strain relationships and make it difficult for mothers to engage in parenting and household responsibilities. Addressing postpartum depression can help improve family dynamics and create a more positive and supportive environment for both mothers and their families.

- Economic costs: Postpartum depression can also have economic costs, including increased healthcare costs and lost productivity. By addressing postpartum depression early on, healthcare costs can be reduced and mothers can return to work and other activities more quickly.

- Mental health stigma: Addressing postpartum depression can also help reduce the stigma surrounding mental health issues, particularly among new mothers. By speaking openly about postpartum depression and the importance of seeking help, we can help reduce feelings of shame and isolation and create a more supportive and compassionate society.

Overall, addressing postpartum depression is important for the health and wellbeing of mothers, infants, families, and society as a whole. By increasing awareness, promoting early detection and intervention, and providing effective treatment and support, we can help ensure that all mothers have the opportunity to thrive and lead fulfilling lives with their families.

Future directions for research and advocacy

- Prevention: While there are several effective treatment options for postpartum depression, more research is needed on prevention strategies. Identifying risk factors and developing targeted interventions can help prevent postpartum depression from occurring in the first place.

- Access to care: Improving access to care is critical for addressing postpartum depression. This includes increasing awareness among healthcare providers and the general public, as well as addressing structural barriers to care such as lack of insurance coverage and limited availability of mental health services.

- Cultural considerations: Postpartum depression affects women from all cultural backgrounds, but there may be unique cultural factors that impact how women experience and seek help for postpartum depression. More research is needed to understand these factors and develop culturally sensitive interventions.

- Long-term outcomes: While much research has focused on the short-term effects of postpartum depression, there is a need for more research on the long-term outcomes for mothers and their families. This includes understanding the impact of postpartum depression on child development and family functioning over time.

Advocacy and policy: Advocacy and policy efforts are critical for increasing awareness, improving access to care, and reducing stigma surrounding postpartum depression. This includes advocating for increased funding for research and mental health services, as well as promoting policies that support maternal and infant health and wellbeing.

By focusing on these areas, we can continue to improve our understanding of postpartum depression and develop effective interventions that support the health and wellbeing of mothers, infants, and families.

www.ingramcontent.com/pod-product-compliance
Lightning Source LLC
Chambersburg PA
CBHW071112220526
45467CB00004B/1826